PLAYING WITH MATCHES

Thoughts on Applying to Residency

Gabriella Schmuter, M.D.

Copyright © 2024 Gabriella Schmuter, M.D.
All rights reserved.
ISBN: 979-8-34-452613-3

TABLE OF CONTENTS

5	Introduction
10	Chapter 1: Gaining Perspectives
15	Chapter 2: Picking a Specialty
22	Chapter 3: Setting Goals
28	Chapter 4: Leveraging Your Unique Value
33	Chapter 5: Mentorship
39	Chapter 6: Grades and Rotations
46	Chapter 7: Extracurricular Activities
52	Chapter 8: Research and Publications
63	Chapter 9: The Illusion of Time
69	Chapter 10: Putting It All Together
77	Conclusion
80	References
83	Acknowledgments
84	About the Author

INTRODUCTION

While I don't claim to be an expert on the topic of applying to medical or surgical residencies and I don't have all the answers, I've walked the path. When applying for an ophthalmology residency, I encountered challenges faced by many applicants, especially when there are limited resources for accessing clinical research opportunities or mentorship. I wrote this book as a guide for medical students planning to apply to residency and looking for practical advice, reassurance, and insights from real experience.

My journey began in an accelerated, combined medical program in New York City. This was a tumultuous period in my personal life, and I was reeling from personal loss and emotional upheaval. While searching for a way to channel my energy productively, I discovered a deep appreciation for ophthalmology. Having narrowed my focus, I soon grew intimidated by the daunting statistics and competitiveness of the specialty. Applying to a competitive specialty like ophthalmology presented its own distinct challenges, particularly in finding guidance, opportunities for research, and expert advice on the application process. But over the next four years, with the support of key mentors and colleagues,

I was able to shape an application that reflected my commitment to the field.

As I developed confidence and clarity in my application, I found that the journey itself was transformative. I learned to carve my path by building relationships, writing papers, and accumulating the necessary components—and I successfully applied and matched into an ophthalmology program.

Since then, many students facing similar challenges have come to me with questions. How do you build connections in a field when you have limited access and resources to that specialty? How do you secure meaningful research experiences? How do you stand out in such a competitive environment? While I have always enjoyed sharing my experiences with other students, I found it difficult to cover everything I wanted to say in a single conversation. That's why I decided to write this book.

I hope to offer insights, strategies, and encouragement for those navigating the competitive application process. While my story is framed around ophthalmology, the principles discussed in this book can apply to many other specialties and provide a roadmap for those coming from various schools and backgrounds.

Whether you're just starting medical school or already approaching the application cycle, this book will help you clarify your goals, strengthen your application, and feel more confident in your journey. Applying to residency is a formidable endeavor, but there are common experiences and challenges you can prepare for.

As a current ophthalmology resident, my perspective comes from recently undergoing the application process. Though I am not a program director or an academic faculty member, I believe there is great value in hearing from someone who has recently been in your shoes. There are many excellent resources written by experts with decades of experience, but they can feel far removed from the current landscape and challenges of applying to residency today. This book is different, sharing recent experiences and insights.

At many points throughout medical school, I questioned whether my efforts were leading anywhere or if I was simply putting in work that would never pay off. However, by focusing on building strong connections, maximizing my options, and constantly reassessing my goals, I was able to put together an application I felt proud of. I received thirty-one interview invitations from programs across the country. As a rule, I could accept a maximum of eighteen invitations, so I had many options to consider. My journey highlights several universal themes, such as the importance of mentorship, proactive networking, and strategic planning—lessons that apply no matter what field you're pursuing.

This book is not a "one-size-fits-all" guide, and it's certainly not a set of guarantees. But I have distilled my experience into three core principles that I believe are key to success:

1. Start Early
Begin building your profile, connections, and experiences as soon as possible. Even small steps in the early years of medical school can make a big difference. I'll share some tips on how to explore different specialties early on in your medical school years.

2. Take Charge of Your Path
Be proactive in steering your journey, and don't simply "coast" through medical school. Seek

opportunities, forge connections, and actively shape your application. I'll discuss examples such as leveraging cold emails and online platforms to expand your outreach.

3. Work Smarter, Not Harder
Be strategic about the areas you focus on and how you spend your time. Evaluate your unique experiences and strengths to build an effective, high-quality application. I'll advise on protecting your time and making the most of it.

Throughout each chapter in this book, I'll share both the practical steps I took and the mindset that guided me through the uncertainty and challenges of the application process. Some chapters focus on specific aspects, like finding mentors or writing a personal statement, and others offer broader advice for managing time and overcoming self-doubt.

This book is by no means fully comprehensive on the subject of going through medical school and applying to residency. I do not overtly define each stage or part of medical school or the application process. (There are already many excellent books by experienced academicians that dissect each step of the medical school and residency application.) This book serves as more of an adjunct to provide thoughts, tips, and tricks related to the process. Even as application systems shift and new trends emerge, I believe the core ideas will continue to help build the foundation for a strong application.

It's important to note that my experience is only one of many paths you can take when applying for residency, and my situation was not without its advantages. I applied from a program that conferred a Doctor of Medicine degree in the United States, and I did not face challenges that Doctor of Osteopathic Medicine applicants or international medical graduates might encounter (such as differences in licensing exams and competition). Each journey is unique, and what worked for me may need to be adapted to better suit your circumstances.

The chapters are designed to be practical, recognizing that medical students are busy and need actionable advice. I hope that, by the end of this book, you'll feel more equipped to approach the application process with self-assurance and inspiration.

CHAPTER 1: GAINING PERSPECTIVES

"Seek first to understand, then to be understood."
Stephen R. Covey

Before diving into the specifics of applying to residency, it's crucial to first gain an understanding of where you stand and which specialty you want to pursue. When I started my first year of medical school, I felt an underlying sense of fear and uncertainty about the idea that one day, I would need to apply for residency. It was unclear how I would find the mentorship, research, and guidance to succeed. This concern only grew when I began to look at the statistics for particularly competitive specialties, where there were impressively high averages for board scores and research experiences. Such realization made me feel vulnerable, but it also led to the first (and perhaps most important) lesson I'll share in this book: talk to others to gain perspective.

The process of applying to residency (or even medical school) can vary from person to person, both emotionally and logistically. It also depends on factors including prior experiences, research exposure, and personal support systems. Additionally, the way medical students approach their education differs widely; some thrive on in-person lectures and textbooks, while others prefer independent study through question banks and flashcards. Understanding where you stand in this vast landscape starts with gathering perspectives from various sources. During the early phases of your journey—and even as you progress through medical school, residency, and beyond—actively seek out the experiences and advice of others.

Finding Outside Guidance
So where do you begin? One easily accessible resource is the abundance of online media available today: books, video channels, podcasts, and social media pages. There are countless voices sharing their insights on all things related to medical school, application processes, and life in training. However, remember that perspectives can differ, and not all that you hear will apply to your situation. Some advice may resonate deeply, while other recommendations might seem completely out of touch with your reality—and that's okay. Keep in mind that while online resources are helpful, nothing can replace in-person guidance from those who have recently navigated the application process.

When seeking guidance in person, I recommend starting with those who are a few steps ahead of you. Reach out to seniors and residents who have recently gone through the process or are excelling in their training. In particular, seek out those who have successfully matched into your specialty of interest. These individuals have either "done it right" or are currently doing so, and they have the advantage of understanding both your institution and the specifics of your journey. Ideally, they can offer nuanced advice about coursework and clinical rotations, along with unique tips for navigating your medical school environment. They've likely witnessed or experienced missteps and can help you avoid making the same mistakes.

It's important to be grateful for any advice you receive, even if you don't ultimately follow it. The key is to consider each perspective but ultimately make decisions based on what feels right for your unique journey and goals. Think of it like sifting sand to find pearls and diamonds—the valuable insights you collect are precious gems, and the sand is what you let pass through the sieve to reveal them. This approach will serve you well throughout your training and career, as each stage of your journey will bring new challenges and circumstances for growth. Hearing how others have navigated situations similar to yours can be invaluable.

Another key cohort to seek advice from includes academic faculty in your field of interest who are involved in the residency application process. Once I had decided to narrow my focus to ophthalmology, I learned that academic ophthalmologists at teaching hospitals often play roles in selecting applications and interviewing candidates. Even if they aren't program directors, academic faculty can be closely connected to the process and understand what qualities programs are looking for in residents. (Keep in mind that faculty who are far removed from your field of interest or who serve as generalized student advisors might not offer as much targeted guidance.)

Ask yourself how closely involved the person is with the current residency application process and whether they have been in your shoes at some point in their career. If they are well-connected and immersed in the environment of residency applications, their perspective will likely be more insightful.

Private practice physicians can also offer advice, but those who are deeply involved in academia generally have a more direct understanding of the selection process. Don't limit yourself to seeking advice from just physicians. Physician assistants, nurses, technicians, and industry or pharmaceutical representatives often work closely with residents and attendings and can provide a different, valuable perspective on professionalism, networking, and the field as a whole. Everyone you meet can offer pearls of wisdom—professionally or personally—that can contribute to your understanding of the journey ahead.

Critically Evaluating Advice
While you gather advice, it's important to critically evaluate where that advice is coming from. Be cautious about taking guidance on study techniques from senior students who aren't performing well themselves, or advice on applying to ophthalmology from someone far removed from the field. Though this may seem intuitive, you'd be surprised how often people put significant weight on advice from individuals who may not be the most qualified to give it. Similarly, while those outside of medicine may want the best for you, remember that they may not fully understand the nuances of the current application process. As with any advice, listen and then sift through it carefully, keeping only what aligns with your goals. Every conversation, regardless of the outcome, helps shape your understanding and prepares you to make informed decisions as you move forward in your career. The sooner you begin gathering perspectives, the clearer your path will become.

Key Takeaways
- Gather multiple perspectives before making decisions about residency or specialty.
- Everyone's journey is unique, so seek advice from various sources to clarify your own path.
- Advice from seniors and residents in your field is especially valuable.
- Faculty in your specialty, particularly those involved in residency applications, provide helpful insights. Other medical professionals can offer valuable perspectives on the field.
- Evaluate where advice comes from and apply only what aligns with your goals.

CHAPTER 2: PICKING A SPECIALTY

"The best way to predict the future is to create it."
Peter Drucker

When I started medical school, I worried that it would be difficult to match into my desired specialty. I was aware of the overwhelming match statistics of competitive fields, and I'd heard stories of students from prestigious, top-ranked medical schools struggling to match into certain specialties. I knew my journey would be an uphill climb. It was within this context of uncertainty and apprehension that I began a search for the best specialty for me. Fear can be a powerful motivator.

The Challenge of Limited Exposure Opportunities
I first began exploring various specialties through shadowing, which entailed following a physician around a clinical environment and observing. However, I quickly realized that most medical students are not adequately exposed to all possible career options and specialties. For instance, ophthalmology (along with many other smaller specialties), is often underrepresented in medical curricula. The only exposure to ophthalmology

I received in school—outside of my own proactive efforts—was a single lecture that primarily focused on the content needed for board exams. This is a common experience in all medical schools. This is a common issue, with literature highlighting the limited ophthalmology training that most medical students receive.* The result is that many students (and even practicing physicians) feel uncomfortable handling specialty issues due to the lack of exposure. This limited exposure is not a reflection of the importance of smaller specialties in the medical field, but rather a result of curriculum constraints at most institutions.

The underexposure of certain specialties often leads to students discovering these fields by chance, either through serendipitous encounters or personal connections. Many who pursue smaller specialty fields happen to stumble upon them. Some find inspiration from family members or friends in the field. Others may have gained previous work experience as specialized technicians or physician assistants before entering medical school. But for those without such unplanned exposure, the paucity of avenues to encounter smaller fields can be a significant barrier.

This challenge isn't just limited to smaller specialties. Even for broader fields like internal medicine or general surgery, students often don't gain clinical exposure until their core clerkship rotations—usually in the latter half of medical school. It's tough to make a meaningful decision about your future specialty when you're only

---

* Liao, J., Wright, R. R., & Vora, G. K. (2024). The decline of basic ophthalmology in general medical education: A scoping review and recommended potential solutions. *Journal of Medical Education and Curricular Development*, 11, 23821205241245635. https://doi.org/10.1177/23821205241245635

introduced to it late in your medical school journey. By then, if you're interested in a highly competitive specialty, it can be difficult to build a strong application in the limited time before residency applications are due.

Choosing Your Specialty: The Sooner, the Better
Try and decide on a potential specialty as early as possible—even if that decision is just a placeholder. There's nothing wrong with setting a goal in college or early medical school, knowing full well that it may change as you progress. Establishing a goal to work toward a specialty is more important than actually committing to it—at least in the beginning. You can always change your mind later, and the path you choose early on is not set in stone. Medical training is inherently a time of exploration and self-discovery, and changing your specialty interest is completely acceptable, no matter how much time or effort you've invested.

The fear of changing your mind, often driven by the sunk cost fallacy,* is real. The sunk cost fallacy is the idea that you should stick with something just because you've already invested time or effort, even if it no longer feels like the right fit. You may worry that dedicating time to research, shadowing, or networking in one specialty, only to choose another, means that effort was wasted. I argue the opposite. Every experience—whether it's research in a specific specialty, shadowing physicians, or even exploring outside interests—enriches your journey, broadens your perspective, and

---

* Strough, J., Bruine de Bruin, W., Parker, A. M., Karns, T., Lemaster, P., Pichayayothin, N., Delaney, R., & Stoiko, R. (2016). What were they thinking? Reducing sunk-cost bias in a life-span sample. *Psychology and Aging*, 31(7), 724–736. https://doi.org/10.1037/pag0000130

contributes to your growth as both a professional and a person. No time or effort is truly wasted.

Finding Opportunities for Specialized Experience
So how do you choose a specialty early on when you haven't yet been exposed to all the options? There are many resources available that provide overviews of different specialties, from books to online "day in the life" videos on social media. These can be invaluable in helping you understand what a particular specialty entails. Many students choose their specialty based on what aligns with their personality, their preferred work environment, and whether or not they enjoy surgery or procedures. For me, having a mother who was an internist gave me a glimpse into the medical world at a young age. I also read books on the topic, one of which was *The Ultimate Guide to Choosing a Medical Specialty* by Dr. Brian Freeman,[*] which offered detailed descriptions of different fields.

When you're exploring specialties, a fundamental question to consider is whether you see yourself doing procedural or surgical work. I've always been drawn to the idea of mastering a craft with my hands, and I frequently read medical memoirs about surgeons during my middle and high school years. By the time I reached medical school, I found myself considering specialties, including dermatology, otolaryngology, and ophthalmology.

Leverage Contacts for Shadowing Opportunities
With no personal connections in my fields of interest, I reached out to an emergency medicine physician (who was my mother's coworker), and they were able to connect me with an ophthalmologist to shadow for

---

[*] Freeman, B.S. (2013). The Ultimate Guide To Choosing a Medical Specialty (3rd ed.). McGraw-Hill Education.

a few days in the clinic and operating room. This point further highlights the benefit of networking with physicians outside of your specialty of interest. Medicine can be a small world, and many physicians across different fields work closely together. Similarly, I was able to connect with a private practice dermatologist and an otolaryngologist to shadow.

To this day, I greatly value the shadowing experiences I had during my first year of medical school. Shadowing for even just a few days offered me insights into the daily lives and work of these specialists. Each experience was transformative and gave me a window into the unique culture of each specialty. I saw how a dermatologist in private practice could design her office to reflect her personality, control her schedule, and build patient relationships that spanned both medical and cosmetic care. I witnessed the excitement and precision of the operating room while shadowing an otolaryngologist, and my fascination with endoscopic surgery grew as I saw the collaborative, team-based environment that defined this specialty. As you may have guessed, the most impactful moment for me was when I shadowed an ophthalmologist in both the clinic and the operating room. I distinctly remember seeing cataract surgery for the first time and watching the delicate manipulation of tiny ocular structures under magnification, which opened my eyes (quite literally) to the world of ophthalmology. The idea of performing such intricate procedures on a small organ that so greatly impacts patients' lives was awe-inspiring.

Indirect Networking for Shadowing Opportunities
Don't be discouraged if you don't have a relative or acquaintance in medicine who can help you network

with other professionals. Your medical school's administration can help connect you with faculty at affiliated hospitals and any physician you know may have colleagues in your field of interest.

If you have no connections directly or indirectly, then cold emailing can be an effective strategy. Alternatively, networking with others through conferences or specialty organizations can help facilitate shadowing options. Most physicians are very willing to have students shadow them and are often enthusiastic about teaching. While large academic institutions may have strict regulations on who can enter clinical or operating room spaces, private practices or ambulatory surgery centers often have more flexibility and are open to hosting medical students.

Making the Most of Shadowing Experiences
Shadowing does not have to be a long-term commitment to be meaningful. Even a few days of shadowing can provide a deep and informative experience that leaves a lasting impression. During your shadowing experience, remember to be respectful, curious, and grateful. Acknowledge the generosity of the physician and other staff members who welcome you into their space, and always express gratitude to patients who allow you to observe. However, keep in mind that every physician's practice is unique. A single "day in the life" shadowing experience may not be representative of an entire specialty, though it can still give you valuable insight into whether the nature of the work resonates with you.

Ultimately, I felt most drawn to ophthalmology, although I knew that my journey in understanding the specialty was just beginning. I had a goal to work toward and a specialty to continue exploring. And that's what I encourage you to do: explore as early as you can, pick a specialty to focus on and understand that it's okay if you later decide to go in a different direction. It's all part of the process.

Start building connections, gaining experience, and learning about the field. When the time comes to begin applying for residency, you'll be better prepared, more informed, and more confident in your decision, whether you end up sticking with your initial specialty or changing course along the way.

Key Takeaways
- Pick a specialty early, but be open to change.
- Don't fear changing directions.
  Every experience adds value!
- Shadow physicians to gain insights into different specialties.
- Proactively explore underrepresented fields and smaller specialties.
- Leverage connections and networks for shadowing options.
- Be grateful for opportunities and remain open to new experiences.

CHAPTER 3: SETTING GOALS

"Our goals can only be reached through a vehicle of a plan, in which we must fervently believe and upon which we must vigorously act. There is no other route to success."
Pablo Picasso

In my first year of medical school, I set a clear goal for myself to match successfully into ophthalmology. I knew this was ambitious as I encountered the limited resources in the field immediately available to me. I had no research experience in the field, no connections aside from a single shadowing experience, and no mentors to guide me through the process. Realizing these gaps helped me frame the clear goals I needed to set for myself: finding mentors, gaining research experience, succeeding in my classes, and learning all about ophthalmology.

Identifying Gaps in Your Experience
Once you've decided on the specialty you want to pursue, the next step is understanding what it takes to apply successfully and assessing where you currently stand. Each year, the National Resident Matching Program

(NRMP)* and specialty-specific organizations like San Francisco Match (or SF Match, for ophthalmology and urology)** publish match statistics. These include data on board scores, number of publications, and match rates. While it's helpful to sift through these numbers and look for trends, it's important to remember that they only tell part of the story.

As you might expect, competitive specialties with lower match rates often require higher board scores and more research experience. But other critical components aren't as easily captured by statistics. Factors like connections and relationships within the field, the quality of your letters of recommendation, and your personal fit with programs can be just as important. Keep in mind that components like clerkship grades, personal statements, extracurricular activities, leadership roles, previous work experiences, and even academic pedigree can all play a role in crafting a competitive application.

When I first decided to pursue ophthalmology, it was clear where I stood compared to the data: I was starting with essentially nothing. I haven't taken any board exams yet. (Step 1 is typically taken in the second year of medical school, Step 2 in the third year, and Step 3 during residency). I had two undergraduate research experiences—both posters presented at smaller conferences—but little else that would bolster an ophthalmology application. Though I'd been active in leadership roles throughout high school and college, most of those experiences weren't directly relevant or particularly notable when applying to residency. Nevertheless, it's

---

*   National Resident Matching Program. https://www.nrmp.org.
** SF Match. SF Match Residency and Fellowship Matching Services. https://www.sfmatch.org.

important to note that if you have meaningful or transformative experiences from earlier in life, they can still be worth including in your curriculum vitae (CV). For example, I served as school president in high school, a role that shaped my early leadership skills. In college, I participated in student government and committees, which helped build the foundation for leadership roles I would pursue later in medical school. These experiences remained proud parts of my CV.

Building an Application Strategy and Prospective CV
Depending on where you are in your medical training, your goals will vary. If you're starting early—say, in your first year —you have the advantage of being able to plan proactively and can create experiences and skills to align with your chosen field. However, if you're in your second or third year, you may already have some board scores, clerkship grades, and other elements that will shape your application strategy. At this stage, time may become a limiting factor. You may find yourself needing to double down on certain areas, like research or clinical experiences, to bolster other parts of your application that aren't as strong.

The best way to get started is to make a list of what a robust application in your desired specialty requires. Then, assess yourself objectively to see where you stand and what areas need improvement. It can also be helpful to create a "prospective CV," or a document that lists the ideal projects, experiences, and achievements you hope to add to your CV in the coming years. Keep a notebook of thoughts and ideas from a variety of sources—books, social media, online forums, and conversations with others in the field— to keep your information all in one place and help you develop a strategy for your application.

Staying Focused and Motivated

There are several strategies for effective goal setting. One widely used framework is known as the SMART criteria.* This involves creating goals that are Specific, Measurable, Achievable, Relevant, and Time-bound. Incorporating these principles is crucial to avoid setting unrealistic goals that can lead to feelings of defeat. It's also important to structure your goals across different timelines: short-term, medium-term, and long-term. For instance, matching into a specialty might be your overarching long-term goal, supported by smaller, daily or weekly goals that are more readily attainable. As each year of medical school presents new challenges, such as starting core clinical clerkship rotations, your goals should adapt to align with the unique opportunities and requirements of each stage.

Regular self-reflection is also key. Every month or two, take a moment to review which strategies for your goals are working well and which aren't. This practice of periodically evaluating your progress allows you to make necessary adjustments in a timely manner, whether it's prioritizing research options, seeking mentorship, or refining your study habits. This type of regular self-analysis is something I continue to do in both my residency and my personal life. I find it invaluable to reflect on whether or not my daily habits and routines are helping me move toward my goals.

Try drawing inspiration from self-help and psychology books that explore the habits of successful individuals and detail how to implement those habits in your own life. These resources can serve as motivational

---

* Doran, G. T. (1981). There's a S.M.A.R.T. way to write management's goals and objectives. Management Review, 70(11), 35–36.

tools that provide actionable strategies for improving productivity, efficiency, and overall well-being. You might find that integrating the principles of time management, goal setting, and mindset shifts into your daily life can benefit not just your academic performance but your general quality of life during medical school.

Just as personal development goals, fitness aspirations, or New Year's resolutions change, it's natural for the goals and objectives related to your residency application to evolve over time. The key is to be flexible and compassionate with yourself. The process of setting goals is dynamic, and as you gather more information, meet new mentors, and discover doorways for collaboration, your targets will shift. Being open to these changes and understanding that your path may look different from what you initially envisioned is just an important part of the journey.

Less Comparison, More Balance
One of the biggest challenges you may face is the temptation to compare yourself to your peers. Remember, Theodore Roosevelt once said, "Comparison is the thief of joy." It's common to look at your classmates who are applying to the same specialty and measure your progress against theirs. However, focusing on your journey is critical. Your goals should be about *your* growth and transformation, not about surpassing others. Your application journey is a process shared by many talented and diverse students from across the country, each bringing their strengths. Trying to stack yourself against others is often an exercise in futility, and it can be emotionally draining. That said, it can be helpful to take a broader bird's-eye view of where you stand relative to others in your specialty. Doing so in a constructive, practical way

can help you identify areas of improvement and refine your goals, but it should not overshadow your focus on your progress and well-being.

Finally, don't lose sight of your personal goals as you navigate medical school. Prioritize activities like working out, spending time with family and friends, exploring your city, and engaging in hobbies you enjoy. It's easy to become entirely consumed by academic goals, but maintaining a balanced life is crucial for your long-term success and mental health. Your personal goals will help you stay efficient, focused, and resilient without risking burnout.

Key Takeaways
- Understand what your desired specialty requires and assess where you stand.
- Use tools like a prospective CV and SMART goals (Specific, Measurable, Achievable, Relevant, Time-bound) to structure short, medium, and long-term objectives.
- Periodically review your progress, adjust goals as needed, and stay adaptable.
- Focus on your journey rather than comparing yourself to others.
- Maintain personal well-being by prioritizing hobbies, fitness, and relationships to prevent burnout.
- Identify gaps and take actionable steps, such as finding mentors and gaining relevant experience.

CHAPTER 4: LEVERAGING YOUR UNIQUE VALUE

"To be yourself in a world that is constantly trying to make you something else is the greatest accomplishment."
Ralph Waldo Emerson

Each year, application processes appear to become increasingly competitive, whether it's for college, medical school, residency, or fellowships. Today's applicants come from a wide variety of impressive backgrounds, but it's important to remember that your unique path is just as valuable. It's not uncommon to find yourself comparing your experiences to those who have had entire careers prior to medicine or who have taken time off for compelling research projects or international experiences.

The key part of the application journey is discovering your own story—how you became who you are and what brought you to this point. You may already feel confident in the narrative you've shaped through your interests, hobbies, and passions, or you may still be figuring it out. Either way, medical school itself is a period of significant personal and professional growth; simply navigating its demands is transformational.

Defining Your Personal Story and Potential

Part of the residency application process involves crafting a personal statement and being prepared to share your story. One common interview question is, "Tell me about yourself." In these moments, your challenge is to convey, in just a couple of minutes, why you are a compelling applicant and a good fit for the program. Think of it as your "elevator pitch," where you present your value and story in the time it takes for a brief elevator ride. This can be difficult if you're still undecided about your specialty or struggling to stay afloat in the demanding environment of medical school.

Your story will evolve throughout medical school as you encounter a wide range of adventures. I recommend immersing yourself as fully as possible in what makes up the "medical school experience" and embracing its challenges, opportunities, and unique moments of growth. Every student has a unique story that brought them to medicine, whether it's a personal encounter with the healthcare system or working with someone who inspired them. When it comes to applying for residency, programs will want to know not just why you chose medicine but why you are passionate about a specific specialty. Reflect on what sets you apart—your background, experiences, challenges, and mentors—and use these elements to craft a narrative that highlights the value you bring to a program.

This perspective is crucial: recognizing that you have something valuable to offer the residency program for which you're applying. It's easy to feel small and overwhelmed in the competitive application process, but confidence in your hard work and preparation can set you apart. This confidence isn't arrogance or hubris; rather, it's the assurance that your dedication and unique perspective have prepared you to contribute meaningfully. This self-assuredness will be evident in your statement, your interviews, and in every interaction with faculty. It stems from building a thoughtful, compelling application that reflects your genuine interest and commitment to the field. If you've put in the work through research, strong academic performance, and meaningful experiences, you can be confident in the value you bring to a program.

Creating an Honest and Compelling Application
An application doesn't need to be "perfect" to be compelling. If there are gaps, setbacks, or elements of your story that might seem like "red flags," embrace them. Acknowledging and growing from challenges demonstrates resilience and self-awareness. For example, when the United States Medical Licensing Examination (USMLE) Step 1 was scored (before the pass/fail change in 2022), a strong Step 2 performance was often a way to demonstrate improvement. If certain grades didn't turn out as well as you hoped, you had a chance to show a wealth of research or clinical experiences. Resist the urge to fit yourself into a predefined mold. Your unique personality, interests, and life goals are what set you apart.

During my application process, a central theme in my story was the limited resources directly available to pursue ophthalmology, and I shared how I carved my path by seeking opportunities in the surrounding city. I also discussed my hobbies—traveling, skiing, trying new restaurants (I even had an amateur restaurant review blog at one point), and collecting shoes—which contribute to who I am outside of medicine. These interests make you memorable, relatable, and contribute to the overall culture and camaraderie of the residency program. I shared my upbringing as a first-generation American, the child of parents who emigrated from the former Soviet Union. My mother's journey—which included repeating medical school twice (once in Belarus and again in the United States) to become a practicing physician—was a significant inspiration for my path in medicine. I also spoke about my incredible mentors, who gave me chances to improve and encouraged my pursuit of ophthalmology.

Realizing early on that medical school is a time for learning, growth, and becoming the best version of yourself can help frame your experiences. By the time you reach the end of medical school, your story will have naturally come together, reflecting both your journey through medicine and who you are as a person. Keeping in mind that one day you'll need to write a personal statement and share this story can help you stay mindful and intentional throughout your years in medical school. Embrace the journey, reflect on your growth, and your unique value will shine through.

Key Takeaways
- Your background, experiences, and challenges make you stand out; use them to craft a compelling narrative.
- Be assured of the hard work and preparation you've put in, and show confidence in your application and interviews.
- Address setbacks openly, showing resilience and growth instead of imperfections.

- Mention your hobbies and the unique aspects of your personality, which make you memorable and contribute to residency program culture.
- Recognize that medical school is a time of personal development and learning, and use these experiences to shape your story for residency applications.

CHAPTER 5: MENTORSHIP

"What you leave behind is not what is engraved in stone monuments, but what is woven into the lives of others."
Pericles

Relationships are at the heart of the medical field—they provide support and meaning to our experiences. The medical field provides an incredible opportunity to connect with people from all walks of life, both as colleagues and patients.

Mentorship, as I see it, is a professional relationship with someone (typically in a more senior position) who has achieved or is pursuing goals that align with your own. These relationships can take many forms and land anywhere along the spectrum of formality. You can have numerous mentors, each serving different purposes in terms of providing career advice, research advice, or advice for navigating and balancing your personal life alongside the demands of medicine. Just as a mentor's role is to guide, a mentee's role is to be proactive, respectful, and engaged. The relationship is a partnership, with both sides contributing to mutual growth and success. Furthermore, professional mentorship spans generations; our mentors and mentees eventually become our colleagues. It's a unique relationship that underscores how much we need one another to succeed in this field.

In medical school, students often seek mentors for advice on navigating their education, applying to residency programs, and collaborating on research. While mentors are often established faculty, they can also be peers—students or residents just a few steps ahead, or even in different fields.

Connecting with Potential Mentors

When I decided early in medical school to pursue ophthalmology, I quickly realized the importance of connections in such a small specialty. Initially, I faced a challenge: I was passionate about ophthalmology but had no direct way to meet people in the field. While I had family in medicine, none were ophthalmologists, nor did we have close friends or coworkers in the specialty. While existing personal connections can provide an initial advantage, seeking out opportunities with initiative can be equally effective in building the necessary relationships for success. If you're fortunate to have a robust department in the field of your interest at your medical school, reaching out to faculty, coordinators, or program directors can be invaluable. At institutions with strong departments, there are often ample prospects for mentorship, clinical exposure, and research. But what if your medical school has limited resources in the field of your interest?

Sending Effective Cold Emails

Being in New York City meant that I was surrounded by many world-class institutions and teaching hospitals. I began cold-emailing various ophthalmologists in the city who I did not know, seeking a research mentor. My emails were concise and tailored: I introduced myself as a first-year student eager to learn about ophthalmology and willing to commit to research projects throughout medical school. Attaching a CV, however modest, was crucial, as was highlighting any shared research interests to make my email stand out.

Cold emailing can be daunting, especially since you're reaching out to busy academic physicians who juggle clinical work, administrative duties, and their personal lives, all while mentoring students at their own institutions. I viewed these emails as an "elevator pitch": a brief (yet persuasive) message that conveyed why they should consider my proposal and offer an opportunity. Conciseness is key, as is understanding the recipient's perspective.

Even with a well-crafted email, be prepared for no response or polite refusals. Persistence is vital. To keep track of my efforts, I used a spreadsheet to log the details of each contact: names, subspecialties, affiliations, dates of contact, responses (yes, no, maybe), and any follow-ups. Ultimately, I reached out to around thirty-five ophthalmologists over a few weeks, received many non-responses, a few "maybes," and one invaluable "yes."

In-Person Networking
Medical conferences are fantastic for meeting potential mentors, sharing research, and staying current with developments in the field. From smaller local gatherings to large national and international meetings, these events provide opportunities to build relationships, share your interests, and explore collaboration. I've found the more intimate settings of smaller conferences (typically local

or regional events, or conferences affiliated with an organization that has a smaller membership volume) make them especially conducive to forming deep connections. Additionally, social events such as mixers, dinners, or grand rounds offer more casual environments to build rapport and discuss ideas with potential mentors and colleagues.

Mentors you meet at in-person events may work at institutions that are geographically far away from you, which can complicate collaboration. However, social media platforms allow you to connect with physicians, follow their work, and engage in discussions that can lead to long-distance, virtual mentorship. (I discuss some details of my experience with social media and finding mentorship as a medical student in a brief editorial as referenced.[*]) Numerous organizations also offer webinars and mentorship programs online, expanding opportunities to connect and learn remotely.

Even in a small specialty like ophthalmology, a single connection can have a domino effect, leading to many more introductions. For instance, research mentors often have a group of residents, fellows, and students who will become part of your network. Similarly, colleagues in other fields can introduce you to relevant mentors in your specialty.

Becoming a Mentor
Just as important as finding mentors is becoming one. Sharing your knowledge and experiences not only supports the next generation but also deepens your under-

[*] Schmuter G, Tooley AA, Chen RWS, Law JC. Social Media in Ophthalmology: The Educational and Professional Potential for Medical Students. J Acad Ophthalmol. 2020;12(1):e41-e45. doi:10.1055/s-0040-1709178.

standing and builds lasting friendships. As a resident, I now enjoy mentoring medical students and collaborating on projects. Working together allows everyone involved to leverage their distinct strengths. While I may have less time for labor-intensive projects (such as those that involved chart review) during residency, students often have more flexibility and availability in their schedules to participate, making collaboration mutually beneficial.

The single "yes" I received from my cold emails opened the door to a mentorship that became the catalyst for my profound journey into ophthalmology (with a focus on oculoplastic surgery). That initial connection with two fellows in oculoplastics introduced me to a dynamic and tightly-knit community of researchers, educators, and clinicians within ophthalmology. As I delved deeper into this world, I met residents, fellows, and faculty whose guidance shaped both my professional path and my personal growth. These mentors offered more than just knowledge or opportunities—they helped mold my understanding and appreciation of meaningful relationships in medicine.

The most striking part of my journey has been watching one oculoplastic fellow who mentored me in those early days rise to become my program director. It's a humbling reminder of the cyclical nature of mentorship in medicine. The relationships we build, the people we connect with, and the mentors who walk alongside us make this path not only achievable but deeply rewarding.

Key Takeaways
- Success in medicine, especially in competitive fields like ophthalmology, often hinges on finding supportive mentors to guide your journey.

- Take initiative in finding mentors through family, faculty, cold emails, or networking at conferences. Persistence is key.
- You can have different mentors for various aspects of your career, from research to personal growth.
- Being a proactive mentee and later becoming a mentor yourself strengthens relationships and contributes to mutual growth.
- Conferences, social media, and virtual platforms offer avenues to build meaningful mentor relationships, even remotely.
- Relationships in medicine evolve, and those who mentor you may later play key roles in your career.

CHAPTER 6: GRADES AND ROTATIONS

"There are no secrets to success. It is the result of preparation, hard work, and learning from failure."
Colin Powell

Many liken medical school to drinking from a fire hose—the sheer volume of information is relentless, and the pace can be overwhelming. Surviving medical school alone is an impressive feat, but as you progress through your training, you quickly learn there is much more to juggle beyond your coursework. In addition to excelling in classes, there are pressures to engage in research, build professional connections, secure compelling letters of recommendation, and maintain personal well-being. Understandably, students can feel overwhelmed by these demands. Despite the multitude of tasks on your plate, performing well academically and in your rotations is a foundational aspect of building a successful residency application.

When I was preparing to study for classes, I found it invaluable to seek advice from senior students who were excelling—particularly those at my medical school. It is important not to seek advice from just anyone. Focus on those who are achieving what you wish to achieve. Find the students who discovered effective strategies and are excelling on exams and rotations and seek to learn from them. Although medical schools across the United States may differ in ranking and reputation, the core curriculum is fairly standardized due to national licensing requirements. The expectations for the board examinations are the same across the country, meaning that students at different institutions often adopt similar study habits. Online forums, social media channels, and educational online videos can also provide excellent strategies for studying for classes, board exams, and clinical clerkships.

Understanding the Importance of Grading Structure
It's also crucial to understand the specific grading structure of each class and clerkship at your institution. During my time in medical school, my classes in my preclinical years (Years 1 and 2) were generally graded as pass/fail, with the USMLE Step 1 exam holding the most weight. The key for me during those first two years was to study not just for the sake of passing each course but with the long-term goal of mastering content relevant to the forthcoming board examinations. This approach allowed me to build a solid foundation that paid dividends when it came time to prepare for Step 1. By the time core clinical clerkships began, I recognized that our grades were primarily based on clinical evaluations from preceptors, with a smaller portion of the grade coming from the multiple-choice shelf exam. This meant that the bulk of my effort needed to go toward my day-to-day clinical performance. While the shelf exam still mattered,

my focus was on excelling in my clinical duties, engaging in patient care, and working well with my team.

Be efficient with your time and strategically allocate your efforts toward what holds the most weight in your evaluations. If your clinical performance accounts for the majority of your grade in a clinical rotation, then focus on making each day count when in the clinic or operating room. On the other hand, if a shelf exam or standardized test carries more weight, adjust your study habits accordingly. Efficiency is crucial, and you don't want to spend excessive time on material that isn't likely to be tested or applied clinically. Use that extra time for other significant elements of your overall application or simply to maintain your well-being and self-care. Success in medical school involves balancing academic performance alongside your physical and mental health.

Regardless of any changes that arise in your institution's policies for tests and grading, and no matter how national standards shift, staying informed about which exams are the most important will help you align your study habits and time management effectively. The abundance of dense textbooks and study materials in medical school can easily lead you down a rabbit hole, so staying focused on what is most likely to be tested on exams (frequently referred to as "high yield" information) is critical.

Developing Study Strategies
Be honest with yourself about your learning style, and remember that not everyone learns in the same way. Struggling in medical school often has more to do with using the wrong study techniques or timelines rather than an intrinsic inability to master the material. Some students thrive with flashcards and question banks,

which are effective tools for memorizing minutiae for exams. Others find that live lectures and textbooks are more helpful. Whether you are someone who benefits from a classroom setting or prefers independent study, there is no "right" way to learn—it's about what works for you.

I found that independent study with flashcards and question banks was the most effective study technique for me. Knowing this, I was able to study more efficiently and allocate extra time for exercise, extracurriculars, research, and other activities that were important to me. The ability to maximize your efficiency is key to balancing the demands of medical school. It is a great achievement to determine a learning method that works for you and allows you to find balance in your life.

When it comes to studying for the USMLE board exams, it's never too early to start. The breadth of material covered is extensive, and integrating your board preparation with your preclinical studies helps to solidify key concepts early on. It is also important to consider that classroom-based learning typically offers more flexibility and free time than clerkship rotations, where you're often in the hospital all day while still needing to study for shelf exams. Many classroom lectures today are recorded or virtual, giving you the option to tailor your study approach. If live lectures don't suit your learning style, there's nothing wrong with that. Use the format that suits you best to maximize your learning and efficiency.

Succeeding in Clinical Clerkship Rotations

Clinical clerkship rotations are often highly performance-based and vary widely between institutions and specialties. Often, core clerkship rotations (as well as audition or elective rotations in your final year) are looking for students who demonstrate motivation and a strong work ethic. Here are some helpful tips to remember:

- Demonstrate hard work hard each day. Arrive early, stay late when appropriate, and maintain a friendly, team-oriented approach.
- Always be on the lookout for opportunities to help, no matter how small the task may seem. This builds trust and respect from your team.
- Appear interested and engaged. Dress sharp, be professional and enthusiastic, and introduce yourself to others.
- Ask for feedback early in the rotation. This allows you time to make any necessary improvements rather than waiting until it's too late.

During rotations, you may also have opportunities to engage in case reports or clinical projects. Participation in these activities demonstrate initiative and can also be added to your CV. Any small tasks that may make days easier for your colleagues, residents, and others are appreciated by your team and can help you stand out. Be direct when asking faculty what they expect of you on the rotation and ask for tips to help you succeed. This guidance helped me score honors on all my graded clinical clerkship rotations, even though I wasn't necessarily the strongest student in the cohort in terms of clinical knowledge and academics.

Your clerkship years are an incredibly rewarding time in your training. While they are busy and demanding, they provide opportunities to build meaningful patient relationships and to grow clinically. As medical students often have more time to spend with patients than residents or attendings, you can get to know patients' stories and learn from their experiences. Since rotations can vary in structure and expectations, try to contact senior students, residents, or peers before starting a rotation to receive more personalized advice on how to excel.

Balancing Multiple Rotations
When determining how many audition or elective rotations to do before applying to residency, there is much to consider. Keep in mind that doing more than three elective rotations can be draining, as it places you in a performative environment for extended periods. If you find yourself needing to decline an elective rotation, don't worry. There's often a fear that declining an offer may hurt your chances of receiving a residency interview from that program, but in reality, programs are generally very understanding. Make sure your response is polite ,and you provide a clear reason (e.g., scheduling conflict). As long as you communicate respectfully and with gratitude, it should not negatively impact your application. Most programs understand that scheduling conflicts arise and that medical students are balancing multiple rotations and opportunities at once. The key is to be cordial, transparent, and reasonable in all your interactions, as professionalism and kindness leave a lasting impression.

Aim to complete an elective at any institution where you can genuinely see yourself going for residency. While an elective rotation doesn't guarantee a residency interview, it can allow you to make a lasting impression on faculty and residents. I did one elective rotation at the institution where I ultimately matched for residency, and the experience was treasured.

If you intend to obtain a letter of recommendation from an elective rotation, plan ahead. Email the specific individuals you want to meet and work with, and be transparent about your goals. Rotation structures differ—some involve working with a different faculty member each day, making it difficult to build rapport, so plan to spend time with one attending if possible.

The journey through medical school is about strategic planning, efficiency, and adaptability. Balance your efforts across academics, clinical skills, and personal well-being. Keep refining your study strategies, stay informed about the demands of your program and the residency landscape, and, most importantly, enjoy the process of growing as a future physician.

Key Takeaways
- Excelling in both coursework and clinical rotations is crucial for a strong residency application.
- Focus your efforts on what counts most in evaluations (clinical performance, exams, etc.)
- Use study techniques that work best for you (e.g., flashcards, question banks, independent study) and integrate board exam prep early.
- Ask for feedback during rotations to improve and adjust in time.
- Be proactive in clinical tasks, show enthusiasm, and engage with patients to build relationships and gain experience.
- Choose electives wisely, aiming for institutions you'd like to join for residency, and plan ahead for building rapport with faculty.
- Communicate respectfully, especially when declining opportunities or requesting recommendations, to leave a lasting positive impression.

CHAPTER 7: EXTRACURRICULAR ACTIVITIES

"Leadership is the capacity to translate vision into reality."
– Warren Bennis

Extracurricular and leadership activities play a valuable role in your residency application by providing a window into your passions, interests, and initiative. While these activities may not be the most critical part of your application, they can become key talking points during interviews and offer evidence of your skills as a communicator, role model, team player, and coordinator. The experiences and skills gained through leadership in medical school transfer seamlessly into your career as a resident and attending physician. Academia is filled with opportunities to collaborate with peers, join educational or administrative committees, and take part in mentoring and teaching. Being part of different clubs and activities exposes you to a variety of personalities, work ethics, and team dynamics, all of which equips you to deal with the variety of different encounters with people you will face when practicing in medicine.

Even if you're not naturally drawn to public speaking or traditional leadership roles, getting involved with organizations that genuinely interest you can help your application stand out.

Finding Organizations that Match Your Interests
Professional organizations often have student membership options. These organizations can be local, regional, national, or even international. Joining them is often free for trainees and can provide enriching experiences that will continue to benefit you in residency and beyond. These groups offer networking, mentorship, research, and leadership roles, and being a member demonstrates your dedication to a particular specialty. I've remained active in several ophthalmology societies I joined as a medical student, and they continue to offer possibilities for connecting with mentors, attending conferences, and enjoying networking in beautiful locales. Being part of such societies also provides a sense of belonging and helps mitigate imposter syndrome, fostering the feeling that you are part of your field's community.

While extracurriculars aligned with your specialty can enhance your application, remember that they don't have to be exclusively within that field. Activities that you are passionate about and can speak on meaningfully add depth to your application. These can range from student government and club involvement to community service, research, and even fellowships. The key is to choose activities you genuinely care about, rather than feel compelled to fill every box on your CV. Engaging in activities just for the sake of having something to list often leads to burnout, and it's usually apparent to interviewers if you're not enthusiastic about your commitments.

Starting Your Own Club and Hosting Events

If your medical school doesn't offer clubs or activities in your field of interest, consider starting one. Creating a special interest group can be a great way to engage with your specialty. You might also host a specific event through an established club, such as a guest speaker session or an interactive wet lab within a surgery or medical special interest group. During my time in medical school, an ophthalmology interest group was founded, opening doors for collaboration, learning, and connection. As a resident, I was later invited back to lead a wet lab dissection to explore the anatomy and pathology of the eye. These activities provide unique opportunities for students, residents, and faculty to learn from one another, build connections, and explore their fields.

Hosting community-based events, such as screening clinics, can be impactful experiences and "quick wins," especially if you have limited time. Specialty screening events (like ophthalmology), whether part of a street fair or standalone clinic, allow students to engage in hands-on activities, provide community care, and explore a specialty firsthand. These types of experiences can serve as initial exposure to a particular field and are great to include on your CV, demonstrating your commitment to both service and clinical skills.

Taking Advantage of Remote Activities

It's also worth noting that leadership and extracurricular activities can take place remotely. With virtual platforms becoming more prevalent, many clubs meet remotely to plan events, host conferences, or coordinate projects. Some larger leadership organizations have global reach, with medical students serving on boards or committees that collaborate nationally or internationally. These virtual prospects enable you to work on impactful projects, build networks, and add unique experiences to your portfolio without being limited by location.

Managing Your Time Effectively
Managing your time effectively is crucial for balancing academic demands with extracurricular commitments. Before taking on any new leadership role, consider the time, energy, and responsibilities required. Ask yourself how frequently the club meets, what your role would entail, and whether the experience is meaningfully worth your time. As you develop leadership skills and become known for your reliability, you'll likely be invited to take on additional responsibilities. Early in your career, being open to such opportunities can be beneficial for growth and exposure, but it's also important to recognize when you are spreading yourself too thin. Taking on too much can not only negatively impact your well-being and academic performance, but it can also diminish your contributions to each role.

Delegation is a helpful skill in leadership and essential to effective time management. Many extracurricular activities operate as a team, with responsibilities quickly becoming concentrated at the top. Learning to delegate tasks effectively to other members of your team reduces your workload and helps empower others to contribute meaningfully. Sharing responsibilities allows the team to function more efficiently and helps develop a culture of collaboration, which is beneficial for everyone involved.

There is no "perfect" number of extracurricular activities you need to be involved in. Whether you choose to dive deeply into a few activities or engage with a variety of clubs, what matters most is that you show commitment, interest, and growth. I often find myself saying yes to various opportunities, but my level of involvement varies based on my interests and role. Depth in one role can demonstrate sustained commitment, while breadth allows you to explore diverse interests.

Building Leadership Skills and Confidence
Leadership comes in many forms. Whether you are organizing events, mentoring peers, or contributing quietly behind the scenes, these roles demonstrate important skills like initiative and reliability. Your growth within a leadership role is also important. For instance, starting as a general member and advancing to treasurer, secretary, or president over time reflects dedication and progression, which can stand out on your CV. This visible development underscores your growing experience and engagement.

During interviews, you will likely be asked about your extracurricular activities. It's crucial to include those experiences on your CV and to be prepared to discuss them confidently. Providing a brief description or bullet points on your CV summarizing your key contributions will help remind you of your impact and serve as a prompt for interview discussions.

Embracing Your Unique Hobbies
Hobbies also play an essential role in life and can serve as a point of discussion in the residency application process. I've often met students who feel uneasy when asked about hobbies because they believe they don't have any, but hobbies come in all shapes and sizes. Anything from sports to traveling to arts and crafts, or even fitness, can be hobbies. Interestingly, some hobbies can even subtly align with the nature of your specialty.

For instance, activities requiring fine motor skills (like drawing or painting) might complement surgical interests. Interviewers often comment on your unique interests, and it provides an opportunity to connect on a personal level and show that you're a well-rounded individual with interests beyond medicine.

Key Takeaways
- Leadership roles and activities highlight your passions, teamwork, and initiative, becoming valuable talking points in interviews.
- Engage in activities you're passionate about, whether aligned with your specialty or personal interests, to avoid burnout and demonstrate authenticity.
- If no club exists for your specialty at your institution, consider starting one or hosting events to engage with others and showcase leadership.
- Manage your time wisely and delegate tasks to avoid spreading yourself too thin while fostering collaboration.
- Personal interests and hobbies, even unrelated to medicine, help connect with interviewers and show you're a well-rounded individual.

CHAPTER 8: RESEARCH AND PUBLICATIONS

"The more I read, the more I acquire, the more certain I am that I know nothing."
Voltaire

Research and publications present some of the greatest challenges in medical school, particularly when it comes to getting started. Finding research opportunities and projects can be daunting, especially if your institution lacks robust clinical research prospects or if you don't have a department in the field of your interest (with faculty actively involved in research). For many students, this obstacle is compounded by an uncertainty of how to approach research in a purposeful way.

First, determine whether research is a necessary part of applying into your desired field. One way to do this is by looking at match statistics, which are released annually online and often include a breakdown of how many research experiences and publications the average applicant has. These statistics can sometimes feel overwhelming to look at. Keep in mind that many applicants accumulate these numbers through gap years or during time taken off before, during, or after medical school. Remember, you don't need to match those numbers, but knowing the general expectations for your field is a good starting point.

A related question to ask yourself is what kinds of research interest to you, if any. If you're just starting medical school, it's normal not to have clear research interests yet. When I first decided to pursue ophthalmology in my first semester, I didn't have specific research goals either. My interests evolved, and it wasn't until later that I became more focused on oculoplastics and medical education. Over time, you will naturally discover the areas that interest you the most. It's also entirely possible that you may not particularly enjoy research—and that's okay, too. You may still need to engage in research for your application and to demonstrate your commitment to the field, but it doesn't have to define your future career.

Finding a research mentor is a good step to take, but how much this matters can vary by specialty. Some specialties, like ophthalmology and dermatology, are more research-oriented, and applicants must have research experiences and publications listed on their CVs. For other specialties, it may not be as critical. Nonetheless, research remains a valuable experience for all medical students regardless of what field they apply to, and the foundation of evidence-based medicine.

Finding Research Opportunities

When looking for research opportunities, you'll find that there are several types of research in any given field, including clinical research, bench research (which takes place in a laboratory), and translational research (which bridges the gap between basic science and clinical practice). Most medical students, due to time constraints, tend to participate in clinical research unless they are on an MD/PhD track that focuses more on laboratory-based research. If you are at an academic institution with a department in your field of interest, you may have direct access to clinicians and researchers with ongoing projects. These faculty members can serve as mentors, and by demonstrating your dedication and work ethic, you can develop impactful professional relationships that can open doors to more research opportunities. Building such relationships early on is beneficial in academic research.

Today's digital world offers more options than ever to engage in research remotely. Many specialties have large online databases that are publicly accessible or available through institutional subscriptions. These databases are a great way to engage in research, especially for students without direct access to research prospects at their own institutions. Social media, online communities, and national specialty organizations are also valuable resources for finding research projects and collaborators. These opportunities allow you to work on research remotely and at your own pace without needing to physically be in a lab or clinic.

Residents and fellows can also be great sources for research opportunities. Many residents are involved in research projects but have limited time for tasks like data collection or initial manuscript drafting. Medical students, on the other hand, often have more flexible schedules and can assist with these roles. When it comes time to apply for residency, the residents and fellows you worked with will remember the effort you put into these projects.

While it's ideal to have research experience in the field you plan to apply for residency in, any research experience is better than none. I still list my early research in fields like neurology and immunology on my CV, even though they aren't directly related to ophthalmology. These experiences were valuable and taught me important research skills, so they're still worth including.

Networking Through Research

Research publications and presentations are excellent ways to meet new colleagues, network, and coordinate on future undertakings. At conferences, it's not uncommon to meet others who are interested in working jointly on new projects or providing valuable input on your work. If you are the first author on a project, this can be a great time to take the lead in discussions and drive forward new ideas. I've had success by directly emailing ophthalmologists (even those I had never met in person) whose work I admired, often with the hope to team up on a new idea for a written piece. This has led to substantive teamwork and even helped when applying to residency programs at their institutions. In this way, research can serve as a powerful tool for creating professional opportunities that may extend across the globe.

If your institution lacks a department in your chosen field or has limited research prospects, don't be discouraged. Cold emailing potential mentors at nearby institutions or geographically distant institutions can be a useful strategy for finding research options. (See Chapter 5 for tips on cold emailing.) Similarly, summer breaks and vacations, if needed, can offer time to engage in research, particularly if you're willing to travel to another institution. These breaks may also offer an opportunity to engage in traditional laboratory-based research, which often requires a more significant time commitment. Even if you prefer clinical research, participating in different types of research helps broaden your understanding of medicine and may help you discover new aspects you enjoy.

In many research groups, a combination of residents, fellows, and medical students work together under the guidance of senior faculty. These groups often have several ongoing projects at different stages, allowing you to choose the type of work that interests you most or fits best with your available time. These opportunities to collaborate on multiple projects can be especially helpful for building your research portfolio.

Time Management and Juggling Multiple Projects
The amount of time you have available to devote to research will fluctuate throughout medical school. During my first two years, I had more time for larger projects, like retrospective chart reviews. However, as I moved into clinical clerkship and began spending long hours in the hospital, it became more difficult to engage in time-consuming research projects. Matching the size and complexity of a research project to the amount of time you have available is key to avoiding burnout.

Some research tasks (like chart reviews) can be tedious, time-intensive, and, frankly, a bit boring. I spent many weekends during my first year scrolling through paper charts to collect data for a spreadsheet. It's important to stay focused on the end goal. Listen to music or experiment with ways to stay entertained during tedious activities. Breaking down tasks into smaller, more manageable pieces also helps. You can also allocate specific periods of time for research tasks, such as setting aside two hours for chart review, to make the process more manageable and prevent feeling overwhelmed.

Some institutions offer dedicated research blocks for students, which is an excellent and thoughtful gift in today's competitive residency application era. My institution (like many) did not offer a dedicated research block, so I had to find ways to balance research with my other responsibilities. This requires careful time management, but it's absolutely doable with the right mindset and strategies.

As I became more comfortable with participating in projects, I found myself involved in more and more undertakings—sometimes over ten at a time. While this can be exciting and fun, it can also be quite intense. I often felt like I was behind on all of my projects because as soon as I caught up on one, I fell behind on another. That said, I genuinely enjoyed being involved in multiple projects and seeing them through to completion.

Publication Options and Opportunities

Research publications come in many forms. Beyond traditional clinical research, publications can include editorials, opinion pieces, letters to the editor, and even books or book chapters. If you enjoy writing, these alternative forms of publications offer great opportunities to express your thoughts and ideas while adding to your CV.

Choosing where to submit your research can be tricky, and it's common to receive rejections—sometimes multiple rejections—before your work is accepted. Speaking with faculty and colleagues in your field can help you decide which journals or conferences to target. Reading articles from potential journals and attending conferences can also help you get a sense of the types of research they typically accept. Sometimes, even if your research is primarily in one field, it may be more suitable for publication in a related specialty journal.

In addition to traditional publications, alternative forms of content, such as podcasts or multimedia, can be valuable additions to your CV. Although podcasts are not typically considered formal publications, they showcase your ability to communicate and engage with an audience. I participated in a few podcasts during medical school, where I discussed my experiences and perspectives as a student. I listed these podcasts on my CV, along with links to the episodes, to demonstrate my comfort with public speaking and my willingness to share my experiences with others.

Medical students sometimes think that their opinions aren't valued because of the junior level of their training, but I've found that this isn't the case. In fact, medical students often have particularly valuable insights, especially when it comes to topics such as medical education, where their experience is directly relevant. If you have an interesting idea for an editorial or opinion piece, you can often be the first author—or even the solo author, since it's your original idea. Be confident in sharing your voice and make a unique contribution to your field.

It's possible that, despite your best efforts, you may find yourself in a situation where it's unclear whether your research will lead to a publication or poster that could be listed on your CV. If this happens, it's important to reassess the situation and have an honest conversation with your mentors about your goals. If publication is your goal and it seems unlikely that the project will result in a meaningful end product, it may be time to shift your focus to another project or research group. However, be sure not to burn bridges with your mentor or any colleagues. Every experience is valuable and can teach you imperative lessons about research and collaboration.

To avoid getting stuck in an unproductive research experience, be upfront about your publication goals when you begin working with a research mentor. You can also assess a mentor's productivity by looking up their publication history on medical literature databases. If a mentor hasn't published in several years, that could be an indication that your experience may not lead to a publication or poster. Faculty at academic institutions often have robust resources to engage in research. However, don't discount opportunities with private practice physicians as well, as many have academic affiliations and are highly active in publishing.

Pros and Cons of Taking a "Research Year"
It has become increasingly common for students to take dedicated research time before, during, or after medical school to strengthen their residency applications. Many students choose to take a year (or more) off to focus solely on research. Some students apply for formal one-year fellowships, which have structured programs with clear expectations and deliverables. Many research fellowships offer guaranteed publications or conference presentations based on the number of ongoing projects. Alternatively, students may arrange a more informal "research year" by working directly with a principal investigator.

There are pros and cons to taking time off for a research year. It can be very beneficial and enriching, allowing you to engage in meaningful research projects, collaborate and network with colleagues, travel (for leisure and professional opportunities), and spend time on personal reflection and well-being. That said, taking a research year doesn't always guarantee publications or presentations, especially without the backing from formal fellowships. There are no certainties in research, and the pressure to produce can be stressful. When applicants have taken a research year, there is the natural assumption that the tangible outcomes will be on their CVs. This can raise expectations for students who take a year off, as they may be compared to other applicants who also took research years, and their CVs may be viewed more critically.

The decision to take a research year is a personal one and depends on many factors, including your goals, timeline, and financial situation. Some research fellowships are paid, which may help offset the cost of taking a year off. If it's financially viable for you and you feel that it's helpful for your application, the option is there.

I recommend avoiding time off unless it's necessary. I did not take a research year because I began pursuing ophthalmology in my first year of medical school, which gave me more time to try different research opportunities and accumulate experience throughout the four years. (This contrasts with those who may decide on a specialty later in medical school, particularly toward the end of their third year, when it can be more challenging to gather research experiences in a short amount of time prior to application season.) If your application is strong without a research year, I encourage you to apply without taking the extra time off. Dr. James Dahle thoughtfully considers the potential downside of taking time off in his book, *The White Coat Investor*. He describes the opportunity cost associated with taking time off, particularly that you are foregoing a year of "peak earnings" in the specialty of your choice.*

---

*   Dahle, J. M. (2014). *The White Coat Investor: A Doctor's Guide to Personal Finance and Investing.* White Coat Investor LLC.

If you are not certain about taking a research year, speak with others who have taken time off to get their perspectives. It's important to weigh the pros and cons carefully. It's also common for students who don't match the first time to take a research year to strengthen their application and build additional connections for the next application cycle. Ultimately, whether or not to take time off is a deeply personal choice that depends on your specific circumstances.

When it comes to research, remember to set realistic expectations and avoid overcommitting. The goal should always be to embrace the unique opportunity to contribute to your field, build connections, and develop valuable skills that will serve you throughout your medical career.

Key Takeaways
- Research is more crucial when applying to certain specialties (like ophthalmology and dermatology) but is generally valuable for all.
- Seek out mentors in your field, either through your institution or by cold-emailing faculty, and build connections early.
- Clinical research is often the most feasible for medical students due to time constraints, though bench and translational research are also valuable.
- Begin research as soon as possible to build your CV and connections and be proactive in seeking opportunities.
- Choose research projects that align with the time you have available, especially during busy clerkships.

- For your application, aim for first author roles when possible, though any authorship is beneficial. Not all research experiences result in publications, but the experience itself is valuable.
- Present your work at conferences to build professional relationships and gain feedback.
- Stay focused on meaningful contributions without overcommitting.
- A research year can boost your application, but isn't always necessary. Weigh the pros and cons based on your personal goals and financial situation.

CHAPTER 9: THE ILLUSION OF TIME

"The distinction between the past, present, and future is only a stubbornly persistent illusion."
Albert Einstein

Time flies. We've all heard the saying countless times, but it has never felt more true than during medical school. When you're constantly busy, days blur together, and time seems to accelerate. At first, the residency application process feels like a distant event—but time catches up fast. Even if you start planning your specialty from day one, the application deadline approaches in what feels like the blink of an eye. That's why I'm a firm advocate of starting early. It allows for trial and error, giving you the flexibility to adjust and learn as you go. By starting early, I was able to pace myself, spreading out the various components of the application process across my four years. This allowed me to focus more deeply on different areas without feeling the pressure to rush, even though the passage of time still managed to feel unnervingly fast.

The Benefits of Early Preparation
Preparation isn't just about getting ahead—it's about reducing the inevitable stress. Whether it's studying for boards, drafting personal statements, or gathering recommendation letters, early preparation gives you the luxury of receiving feedback and making meaningful adjustments. Of course, this advice is easier said than done. Medical school is demanding, and it's natural to fall behind or feel exhausted along the way. That's where self-compassion becomes essential. You have to allow yourself the room to fall behind sometimes, to get tired, and to take breaks. Rest is just as critical to your success as hard work, and taking time to recover can help protect your mental health and well-being in the long run.

Setting Your Own Pace
During medical school, I often received critiques from people regarding my intent to begin working quickly on tasks and goals. Some questioned my urgency, saying things like, "You have plenty of time," or "There's no need to rush." But this is where the illusion of time in medical school becomes evident. Deadlines that seem far off approach faster than expected. It's much more comforting to have started early and moved at your own pace than to feel the crushing stress of time running out.

Even with this understanding, losing track of time can happen easily, especially during intense clerkship rotations that keep you in the hospital all day. Procrastination or last-minute cramming become tempting ways to cope. Forgiveness is key during these periods. Allow yourself some grace for not always being on top of everything when you're this busy. But awareness of time's quickening pace is just as important. Don't let things consistently slip through the cracks. Set personal deadlines and pacing to help keep tasks manageable. I've found it helpful to aim to complete assignments a week before their actual due dates, which helps me stay on track when everything around me feels chaotic.

In moments where you feel overwhelmed, grounding strategies become essential. Creating a to-do list or scheduling out tasks can help re-establish some sense of control. Breaking tasks into smaller goals also prevents the overwhelming feeling that time is passing and provides a structure when days mesh together. Other times, it's necessary to take a complete break, disconnect for a bit, and recharge. When you return to work, you will feel refreshed and ready to focus again.

Maximizing Efficiency and Productivity
Using study methods that work best for you—whether that's textbooks, flashcards, question banks, or lectures—can help you manage time more efficiently. This opens up pockets of time that you can use for other important aspects of your life, like self-care, exercise, hobbies, or spending time with family and friends. In medical school, time is your most valuable asset. It's crucial to protect it from distractions or activities that offer little to no benefit. Efficiency is the key to protecting and prioritizing your time.

One challenge I still face, even in residency, is finding uninterrupted time for focused work. I've learned to carve out sections of time (whether early in the morning or late at night) when I can focus intensely on projects or study sessions without the disruptions that fill the daytime hours. Medical school (and residency) can feel like endless cycles of interruptions, so these quiet hours can be immensely productive.

Nurturing an Online Presence

Starting your journey early provides opportunities to build name recognition and your social media presence if you choose to. I'm a strong advocate for using social media professionally as a tool for connecting with others in the field. Throughout my journey, I've shared publications, conference experiences, and personal hobbies and events on my social media platforms. This has helped me build connections with peers, mentors, and colleagues in the ophthalmology community.

That said, it's essential to maintain professionalism, especially when your social media profiles are public. Some physicians prefer to keep their personal and professional lives separate online, while others combine the two. Your reputation, in medical school and beyond, is one of your most important assets. How you interact with patients, colleagues, and faculty—and how you present yourself online—directly impacts how others perceive you and what reputation you will earn. Your reputation often translates into letters of recommendation, reflecting qualities such as your work ethic, reliability, and communication skills. It takes time to build a strong reputation, but it can be destroyed in an instant, which is why it's so important to protect your character both online and in person.

When used wisely, social media is a great way to demonstrate your ongoing projects and accomplishments. By building your online presence early, you can also create opportunities to present at conferences, publish papers, and expand your network—and then demonstrate this publicly via a social media platform. This kind of name recognition can be important during the residency application process and later on in your career.

Protect Your Time—And Your Positivity

Protecting your time also means shielding it from negativity and discouragement. Throughout medical school, I encountered many who doubted my goals or questioned why I was working so hard. Below are some comments I often heard:

> *"You're starting ophthalmology research too early. Relax."*
>
> *"Don't expect to get interviews from competitive programs."*
>
> *"You really shouldn't get your hopes up about ophthalmology."*

These comments weren't said with malicious intent. In fact, many of these people likely felt that they were helping me by giving me a "reality check." However, it is important to distinguish between helpful critiques and unproductive negativity. Staying focused on your goals, even in the face of doubt, is essential. While well-intentioned criticism may have some truth to it, it's important to stay grounded in what feels right for you. Surround yourself with positive influences and environments that support your aspirations. By doing so, you'll not only protect your time but also your focus, happiness, and well-being.

The illusion of time is real in medical school and residency. It's easy to get caught up in the busyness of each day and let time slip by. But by preparing early, protecting your time, and focusing on your goals, you can stay ahead of the curve. Time may fly, but with intention and discipline, you can make the most of every moment and create opportunities for growth, learning, and connection along the way.

Key Takeaways
- Begin preparing for key tasks like research, board prep, and residency applications early to reduce stress and avoid last-minute pressure.
- Use efficient study methods, to-do lists, and personal deadlines to manage time effectively and create space for self-care and personal interests.
- Allow room for breaks when falling behind, as rest is essential for long-term success and mental health.
- Filter out unhelpful negativity and stay grounded in your goals by surrounding yourself with positive influences.
- Consistent professionalism and reliability build a strong reputation over time, which is crucial in medical school and beyond.
- If used wisely, social media can enhance professional networking and name recognition, but maintaining professionalism online is key.

CHAPTER 10: PUTTING IT ALL TOGETHER

*"Everything will be okay in the end.
If it's not okay, then it's not the end."*
John Lennon

Imposter syndrome is a common feeling at every stage of the medical journey, and residency applications are no exception. I remember grappling with feelings of doubt throughout medical school, particularly when pursuing a field that often felt just beyond my reach. One of the best pieces of advice I can offer is to resist the urge to measure your progress against anyone else's and instead focus on your own personal growth. Set goals for yourself and continuously strive to meet your highest potential. There are no guarantees, but you can take control of your journey, doing everything possible to prepare and maximize your chances of success.

It wasn't until the end of my third year that everything began to fall into place. For the first time, I saw how the various pieces of my application, my experiences, and my aspirations were coherently coming together. I finally felt like I had a fair chance and could confidently apply to ophthalmology.

Putting Together Your Application
Before you know it, medical school will come to an end, and you'll face the task of submitting your residency application. All the long hours, exams, and rotations you've endured boil down to this. Start putting together your application early, giving yourself plenty of time to work on critical elements like your personal statement and CV. Ask others to review your materials, too. Sometimes, having an outside perspective can help you refine and polish your application in ways you might not have considered.

As for how many programs to apply to, this varies depending on your specialty and personal circumstances. I applied broadly, submitting applications to around 100 ophthalmology programs across the United States. While this may seem excessive, it helps to cast a wide net in a competitive field to increase your chances of securing enough interviews to make informed decisions. It's better to have more options and later narrow them down than risk not matching because you applied too narrowly.

Lean Into Your Strengths
As you approach the application process, it's important to take stock of your strengths. Medical school has likely revealed what you excel at, whether it's clinical skills, leadership, research, or communication. I learned that my ability to communicate effectively and to lead others were my greatest assets. I also recognized my capacity to maintain a positive attitude and work efficiently under pressure. These were qualities I leaned into as I crafted my application.

Recognizing your strengths not only gives you a clearer sense of what you bring to the table but also boosts your confidence as an applicant. Knowing that you have something valuable to offer helps you see yourself not just as another applicant in a competitive field but as someone with unique contributions to make.

There will undoubtedly be areas where you feel you've fallen short. Maybe you didn't achieve all the goals you set, or perhaps you feel your CV isn't perfect. That's okay. The desire for perfection can sometimes be your greatest obstacle, so focus on the hard work and accomplishments you've accumulated over the years.

Your Personal Statement

Crafting your personal statement can be one of the most challenging and rewarding aspects of the application process. Everyone's story is different, but it's important to stay focused on your own journey within the specialty, not on why you initially chose medicine. By the time you're applying for residency, that broader question has already been answered. Now is the time to focus on what draws you to your specialty and how your experiences have prepared you for it. Give yourself plenty of time to write, edit, and rewrite. Your statement should feel authentic and personal, capturing your unique path.

Letters of Recommendation

When it comes to letters of recommendation, requirements can vary depending on the specialty you're applying to. That said, it's a good idea to keep in mind throughout medical school that you'll need to ask faculty members (typically three) to write strong, supportive letters explaining why you would be an excellent fit for your chosen specialty. Once you've identified your preferred letter writers, ask them well in advance (I recommend at least a month before the submission deadline) to give them plenty of time to write, draft, and follow any upload requirements or guidelines. It can also be helpful to send a gentle reminder a couple of weeks before the letters are due.

Along the way, don't forget the importance of networking and maintaining the connections you've built throughout medical school. There are opportunities to have someone recommend you beyond official letter writing. I reached out to a faculty member I had met only once and politely asked if she might put in a good word for me in her program. To my surprise, she kindly did. It's moments like these that remind you that every connection, no matter how brief, can be valuable. Approach every opportunity with respect and gratitude.

Applicants usually waive the right to view their letters to maintain confidentiality and trust in the process. To assist your letter writers, provide a bullet-point list of specific examples that highlight your character traits, strengths, and any major accomplishments you'd like them to include. You should also share a draft of your personal statement and your CV so they have everything they need to craft a strong recommendation on your behalf.

Residency Interviews
Once the application is submitted, the interview process begins. This can be both thrilling and stressful, so it's important to maintain the routines, habits, and support systems that have carried you this far. When interviews are released, they're often sent via email. It's helpful to set up notifications so you can schedule interviews promptly and secure your preferred dates. With virtual

interviews becoming more common, it's possible to attend interviews in different time zones on the same day, which can be convenient (and challenging). Creating a separate email address specifically for interview notifications was an effective strategy I used, as it ensured I didn't miss any important messages.

Residency interviews, whether in-person or virtual, offer a window into a program's culture, but it can still be difficult to fully differentiate programs based on an interview alone. I found it helpful to connect with current residents outside of the formal interview process to ask more in-depth questions and get a sense of what day-to-day life was really like. If you have the opportunity, doing an away rotation can also give you valuable insight into a program's dynamics, since you'll have the chance to interact directly with faculty and residents over an extended period.

Practice and Prepare Questions
There are many resources online for practicing mock interviews, and I highly encourage taking advantage of them. Whether you're practicing with a senior medical student, resident, or faculty member, mock interviews can help you refine your answers and become more comfortable speaking about your experiences. If your interviews are virtual, consider recording yourself and reviewing the video to critique your performance. This can help you notice any habits you might not be aware of, such as how you appear on camera or the quality of your eye contact.

Also, prepare questions in advance for your interviewers. This demonstrates your interest in the program and allows you to gather information that might not be covered during the interview. Often, interview schedules are sent in advance, giving you the opportunity to research your interviewers. Familiarize yourself with their clinical or research backgrounds to tailor your questions and show genuine engagement.

Interviewing Virtually
The interview process has evolved since the COVID-19 pandemic, with many interviews now taking place virtually. This brings new challenges, from ensuring good lighting and sound quality to presenting a professional background. These details may seem minor, but they can make a difference. Regardless of the platform, the core principles remain the same: be punctual, dress professionally, speak clearly, and be prepared to explain why you're interested in that particular program.

Send Thank-You Emails
After each interview, I recommend sending a brief thank-you email to your interviewers (unless specified otherwise on interview day). This gesture shows appreciation and can help reinforce the connection you made during the interview. The same goes for those who have supported you throughout medical school, such as mentors and letter writers. Notes expressing your gratitude go a long way, and those who have contributed to your success will appreciate the acknowledgment.

Creating Your Residency Rank List
The rank list—arguably the most stressful aspect of this process—requires deep reflection for decision-making. Some mentors may advise that you prioritize program reputation and rank the top programs first. I don't believe there's a one-size-fits-all approach to making a rank list. Instead, focus on what program will be the

best fit for you. Consider elements like subspecialty representation, faculty support, surgical training, and culture. Whether or not you've rotated or done research at a specific program can also impact how comfortable you feel ranking it. Ultimately, you want to end up in a program that has the resources to support your success.

I recommend keeping a spreadsheet during the interview season that documents your impressions of each program. This way, you can go back and organize your thoughts before finalizing your rank list. During my interview season, I experimented with creating an algorithm in my spreadsheet. I assigned weighted values to factors that were most important to me and rated each program based on those factors. This gave me a numerical "score" for each program, which helped me visualize my priorities. While this approach can get technical, it allowed me to see how my gut feelings compared to the logistical details. At the end of the day, rank programs based on what feels most meaningful and right for you.

Match Day
The matching process, as the name of this book implies, is truly like "playing with matches." There are no guarantees, and while there are things you can do to maximize your chances of success, it's still a risky venture. Ultimately, Match Day will arrive, bringing with it a whirlwind of emotions—excitement, nervousness, and sometimes disappointment. Regardless of the outcome, it's important to appreciate the hard work and dedication that brought you to this point.

If you don't match, you're not alone, and there are many paths forward. Some applicants choose to take time off or pursue additional degrees. Others use the time to explore different fields or personal interests. Stay resilient and recognize that not matching is not the end of your journey.

Medicine provides wonderful opportunities that allow us to touch lives in the most profound ways. The journey may be long and challenging, but it all comes together the moment you introduce yourself to a patient as their doctor. That's when the true reward of all your efforts becomes clear.

Key Takeaways
- Focus on personal growth rather than comparing yourself to others.
- Identify your unique strengths (e.g., communication, leadership) and use them to boost confidence as you prepare your application.
- Begin working on your personal statement, CV, and other application components early to avoid stress and allow time for feedback.
- In competitive fields, casting a wide net increases your chances of securing interviews.
- Highlight your story and experiences clearly and authentically, focusing on why you chose your specialty.
- Prepare thoroughly, connect with current residents for more insights, and use mock interviews to practice.
- Consider program culture, faculty support, and personal fit when creating your rank list rather than focusing solely on reputation.
- Utilize the relationships you've built throughout medical school, as every connection can be valuable in the match process.
- If you don't match, remember it's not the end. Many paths forward exist.

CONCLUSION

*"Success is a journey, not a destination.
The doing is often more important than the outcome."*
Arthur Ashe

You can become the physician you aspire to be. You can pursue any specialty you are passionate about. Though the road may be fraught with challenges that are uniquely yours to face, the power to overcome them is within you. Medical school is an extraordinary journey, and to emerge from it is a triumph. It is a victory that demands resilience, sacrifice, and unwavering dedication. Your reward is an opportunity to be part of a profession where care, compassion, and knowledge intertwine to make a real difference.

Don't let your doubt—or the doubts of others—halt your progress. Too often, we second-guess and overthink until what felt within reach becomes impossibly far away. It's this self-imposed limitation that robs so many of their potential, extinguishing dreams before they have a chance to truly ignite. Know this: if you can envision it and commit to the work, you can achieve it.

Reflecting on my own medical school experience, I can now see how I overcame incredible personal challenges. When I began medical school, I was grappling with personal losses that left me feeling defeated and angry. That emotional weight made it difficult to focus, but in time, I channeled my feelings toward a greater purpose. I encountered the field of ophthalmology and turned pain into progress.

Soon after, my medical school experience was marked by the COVID-19 pandemic. I found myself at my parents' house, in lockdown, preparing for the USMLE Step 1 exam. It was a dark time, with the world in turmoil and my future uncertain. My mother, an internal medicine physician, was on the frontlines, treating patients before vaccines were available, and we lived in constant fear for her well-being. Even after I completed the exam, I was mentally drained. Yet, in that space of uncertainty, I learned to endure and to keep moving.

Finally, I arrived at the process of creating my residency rank list. Oddly enough, this was more stressful than the interviews themselves. I wrestled with conflicting advice from mentors, friends, and family, all while trying to reconcile what felt right for me. The permutations of my rank list haunted me, leaving me anxious about the outcome. But, as in every stage of this journey, I learned that it's normal to face unexpected hurdles. It's how we respond—by regrouping, refocusing, and reconnecting with our purpose—that defines our success.

Applying to residency, in many ways, feels like playing with fire. The match process is unpredictable, risky, and full of uncertainty. But while the system has no guarantees, it is your responsibility to maximize your chances. Through it all, never lose sight of who you are. It's tempting to shape yourself into what you think residency programs want, but the only way to truly thrive is by staying true to yourself.

I wish I could reassure my first-year self that all of the stress, the long hours, and the uncertainty will be worth it in the end. The hard work I put in opened doors to opportunities I never imagined were possible. Today, as a resident, I can confidently say I am living the dream I envisioned back then. Residency is demanding, rigorous, and exhausting at times, but it is also deeply fulfilling. I am grateful for the journey, and I know that everything I experienced during medical school—emotionally, mentally, and intellectually—has prepared me for success.

Residency is another stepping stone, and beyond it, the horizon is limitless. In the end, this adventure is about more than becoming a physician—it's about becoming the person you were always meant to be.

REFERENCES

Recommended Additional Reading
- Miller, R. H., & Bissell, D., M.D. (2006). *Med school confidential: A complete guide to the medical school experience: By students, for students.* St. Martin's Griffin.
- Newport, C. (2016). *Deep work: Rules for focused success in a distracted world.* Grand Central Publishing.
- Carnegie, D. (1936). *How to win friends and influence people.* Simon & Schuster.
- Dahle, J. M. (2014). *The white coat investor: A doctor's guide to personal finance and investing.* White Coat Investor LLC.
- Larson, D. (2015). *Medical school 2.0.* Larson Texts.
- Beddingfield, R. (2017). *Med school uncensored: The insider's guide to surviving admissions, exams, residency, and sleepless nights in the call room.* TarcherPerigee.

Quote References

- Covey, S. R. (1989). The 7 habits of highly effective people: Powerful lessons in personal change. Free Press.
- Drucker, P. F. (1994). Managing for the future: The 1990s and beyond. HarperBusiness.
- Pablo Picasso. (n.d.). "Our goals can only be reached through a vehicle of a plan, in which we must fervently believe, and upon which we must vigorously act. There is no other route to success" [Quote]. In BrainyQuote. Retrieved from https://www.brainyquote.com/quotes/pablo_picasso_120939.
- Emerson, R. W. (n.d.). "To be yourself in a world that is constantly trying to make you something else is the greatest accomplishment" [Quote]. In GoodReads. Retrieved from https://www.goodreads.com.
- Pericles. (n.d.). "What you leave behind is not what is engraved in stone monuments, but what is woven into the lives of others" [Quote]. In Goodreads. Retrieved from https://www.goodreads.com.
- Powell, C. (n.d.). "There are no secrets to success. It is the result of preparation, hard work, and learning from failure" [Quote]. In Goodreads. Retrieved from https://www.goodreads.com.
- Bennis, W. (n.d.). "Leadership is the capacity to translate vision into reality" [Quote]. In Goodreads. Retrieved from https://www.goodreads.com.
- Voltaire. (n.d.). "The more I read, the more I acquire, the more certain I am that I know

- nothing" [Quote]. In Goodreads. Retrieved from https://www.goodreads.com.
- Einstein, A. (1955). "The distinction between the past, present, and future is only a stubbornly persistent illusion" [Quote]. In Goodreads. Retrieved from https://www.goodreads.com.
- Lennon, J. (n.d.). "Everything will be okay in the end. If it's not okay, then it's not the end" [Quote]. In Goodreads. Retrieved from https://www.goodreads.com.
- Ashe, A. (n.d.). "Success is a journey, not a destination. The doing is often more important than the outcome" [Quote]. In Goodreads. Retrieved from https://www.goodreads.com.

ACKNOWLEDGEMENTS

Thank you to my parents, Elena Schmuter, DO and Leonid Schmuter. I would like to thank many people who have strongly supported me throughout medical school and residency: Kyle J. Godfrey, MD, Michael Kazim, MD, Andrea Tooley, MD, Gary J. Lelli, MD, Ann Q. Tran, MD, Victoria North, MD, Maria D.L. Garcia, MD, Ronald J. LoPinto, MD, Allison Coombs, DO, Shanlee Stevens, MD, Celestine Gregerson, MD, Bruce Moskowitz, MD, Daniel Garibaldi, MD, and countless others. Thank you to Robert Beale, MD. Thank you to those who reviewed this manuscript and gave input regarding its publication: Ashten Luna Evans, Samuel Pierce, Esq., Alan Samsonov, and Merna Shohdy. Thank you to Natalia Agapova for the wonderful cover design and typesetting.

ABOUT THE AUTHOR

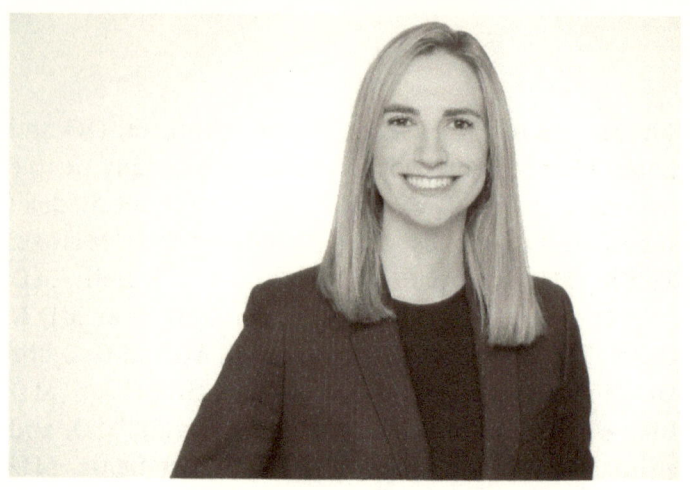

Gabriella Schmuter, MD, is an ophthalmology resident at NewYork-Presbyterian/Weill Cornell Medicine. She earned her Doctor of Medicine degree from The City University of New York School of Medicine, following her Bachelor of Science in Biomedical Science from the Sophie Davis Biomedical Education Program, where she graduated *summa cum laude*. Gabby has published primarily on the topics of oculoplastics and medical education. In her free time, she enjoys traveling, trying new restaurants, collecting shoes, and skiing.

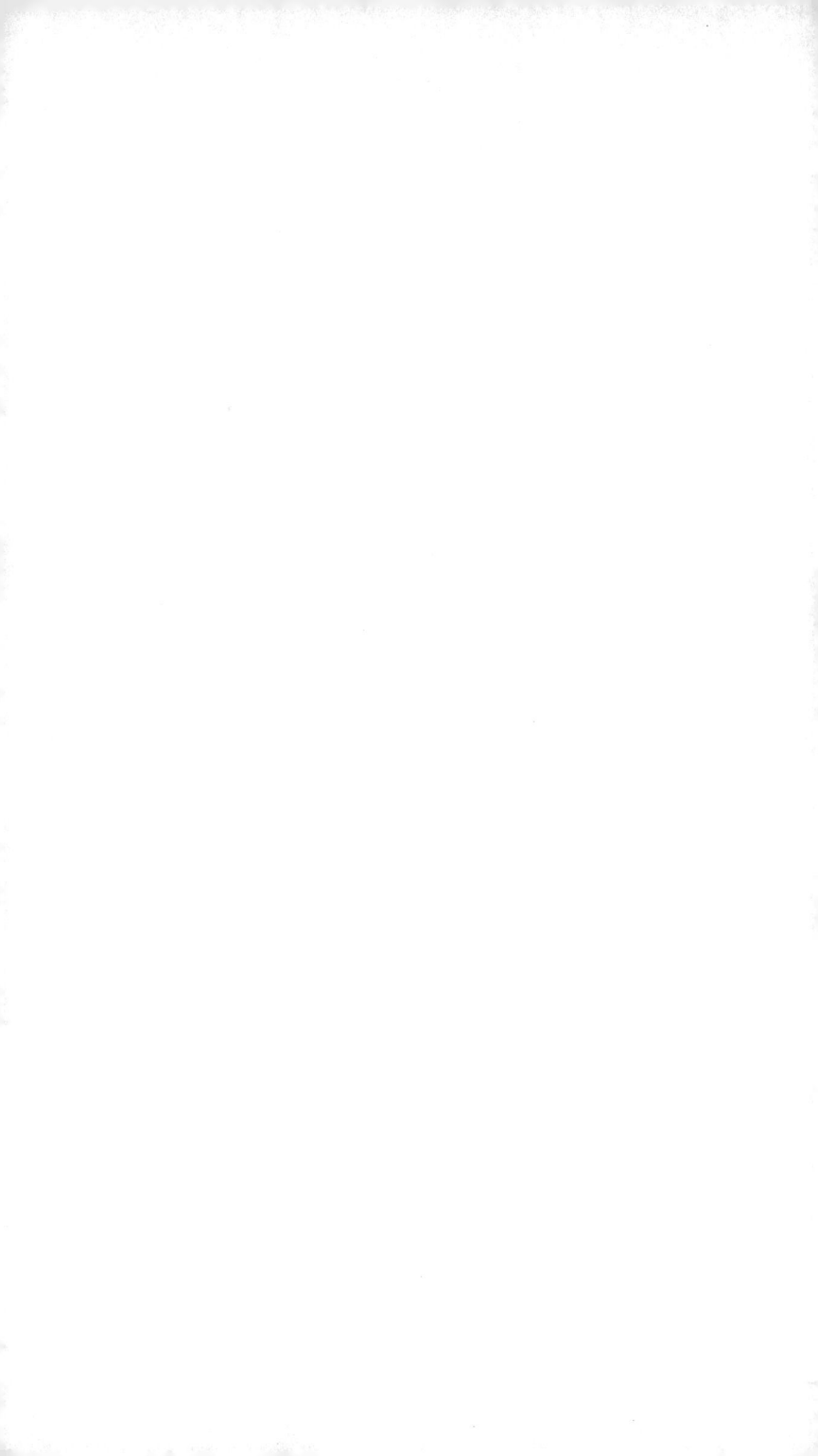

www.ingramcontent.com/pod-product-compliance
Lightning Source LLC
Chambersburg PA
CBHW030447220526
45464CB00006B/2446